YOGA POSES FOR FAST WEIGHT LOSS.

Losing weight and maintaining excellent physical health.

By

Dr DOUGLAS JASON

Before this document is duplicated or reproduced in any manner, the publisher's consent must be gained.

Therefore, the contents within can neither be stored electronically, transferred, nor kept in a database. Neither in part nor in full can the document be copied, scanned, faxed, or retained without approval from the publisher or creator.

TABLE OF CONTENTS

TABLE OF CONTENTS

ABOUT THE AUTHOR

Dr DOUGLAS JASON is a certified dietician who has a strong passion for wellness and a big eagerness to help people all over the world. He uses healthy food, herbs, sauce and other useful tools to help mankind realized it's overall goal of optimum health.

INTRODUCTION

When used in conjunction with a balanced diet, yoga is a powerful tool for losing weight.

Regular yoga practice may also help you relax and enhance your mental health. As a result, people choose their meals more carefully and healthily, thereby contributing to weight reduction.

Having said that, yoga improves your body awareness and relationship with it. You'll be able to choose healthier foods and consume less junk food as a result of this. Yoga has several advantages, some of which are as follows:

greater adaptability
improved respiratory condition
increased vigor and energy
accelerated metabolism
improved physical fitness
higher muscular tone
increased cardiovascular fitness
decrease in weight
stress reduction
Your body and mind may be greatly affected by stress. Pain, worry, sleeplessness, and a lack of focus are just a few ways it may manifest. Stress is often the key factor in weight gain. You may reduce stress by doing yoga.

Losing weight and maintaining excellent physical and mental health are made possible by the physical advantages of yoga and stress management.

The main goals of these yoga postures are to increase body flexibility and muscular tone. Both of these aid in a consistent weight reduction process by increasing the body's ability to burn fat.

CHAPTER 1:

The Plank Pose (Chaturanga Dandasana).

The most effective posture to build core strength is chaturanga dandasana. Despite how simple it seems, it has huge advantages.

Your abdominal muscles don't begin to feel its intensity until you are in the position.

CHAPTER 2

VIRABHADRASANA - WARRIOR POSE.

With the warrior position, it's simpler to tone your thighs and shoulders while also sharpening your focus. The greater the outcomes, the longer you maintain that stance. You may obtain tighter quads by doing Virabhadrasana for only a short while.

Improve your balance while strengthening your back, legs, and arms with the warrior position. If you tighten your abs while maintaining the posture, it will also assist to tone your stomach and give you a flat belly.

CHAPTER 3:

Triangle Pose (Trikonasana)

The trikonasana aids in digestion improvement as well as belly and waist fat reduction. It increases and accelerates blood flow throughout the body. This pose's lateral motion encourages you to lose more belly fat and develop your thighs and hamstrings more. Additionally, it enhances balance and focus.

CHAPTER 4

Adho Mukha Svanasana, or Downward Dog Pose.

Your whole body is toned through Adho Mukha Svanasana, with a little additional focus on certain muscles.

Your arms, legs, hamstrings, and back are all strengthened as a result. Your muscles are engaged and toned as you hold this position while focusing on your breathing, which also enhances your focus and blood circulation.

CHAPTER 5

Sarvangasana - Shoulder Stand Pose.

Sarvangasana has several advantages, including boosting power and improving digestion. It is most well-recognized, though, for increasing metabolism and regulating thyroid levels.

The shoulder stand, also known as Sarvangasana, strengthens the upper body, the abdominal muscles, the legs, and the respiratory system, and encourages sleep.

CHAPTER 6

Setu Bandha Sarvangasana - Bridge position.

The Bridge Pose enhances thyroid function, digestion, hormone regulation, and muscular tone. Additionally, it helps to ease back discomfort by building up your back muscles.

CHAPTER 7

Parivrtta Utkatasana (Twisting Chair Pose)

The yoga equivalent of the squat is known as the Parivrtta Utkatasana. However, you should be aware that it is a bit more vigorous and targets the glutes, quadriceps, and abdominal muscles.

The lymphatic and digestive systems are supported by the asana as well.

CHAPTER 8

Sun Salutation Pose (Surya Namaskara).

The Surya Namaskara, often known as the Sun Salutation, does more than just get the blood flowing and warm the muscles. Most of the main muscles are stretched and toned, the waist is reduced, the arms are toned, the digestive system is stimulated, and the metabolism is balanced.
Since Surya Namaskara focuses on all of your body's core muscles, it provides several advantages.

CHAPTER 9

Power Yoga Pose.

Power yoga is a powerful kind of yoga that revitalizes both the body and the mind.

It is a cardiovascular exercise that increases strength and endurance. Power yoga aids in the maintenance of a healthy body, a stress-free life, and weight reduction. Additionally, it improves mental clarity, flexibility, and stamina.

Power yoga is a contemporary kind of yoga where the asanas build stamina and help you become

strong, flexible, and stress-free. It is
a body-weight exercise that
improves your strength and works
your whole body.

You may benefit from yoga and
more with power yoga positions,
such as
helps to burn calories, somewhat
more so than introductory yoga
It increases metabolism.
It improves your overall health
useful for improving your body's
strength, endurance, flexibility, and
tone.
It enhances your ability to focus.
As tension and stress are greatly
decreased, it aids in your ability to
unwind.

Sun Salutation, also known as
Surya Namaskara, is the first pose
in the most dependable Power Yoga
sequence. Before beginning your
Power Yoga routine, you may warm
up with the Surya Namaskara.

CHAPTER 10

THE 10 BEST POWER YOGA POSES.

The following are some of the top Power Yoga positions for weight loss:
The Wind releasing position, also known as Pawanmuktasana, aids in belly fat loss.
Trikonasana, also known as the posture of intense side stretching, aids in side fat reduction. It increases heart rate and causes calorie burning.
You may lose extra fat from the arms and legs by doing

Dhanurasana, often known as the Bow pose. Body toning is beneficial. For people who desire slimmer thighs, legs, arms, and hands, Garudasana, or the Eagle position, is the ideal option for weight reduction.

Eka Pada Adho Mukha Svanasana, also known as a one-legged downward dog, helps you tone your arms, hands, legs, thighs, and abdominal muscles when done while breathing.

If you want to tone your abs and buttocks, try Bhujangasana, often known as the Cobra posture.

The easiest Power Yoga posture for losing weight is Navasana, often known as the boat pose. It focuses on all of your body's primary muscles.

The most significant posture to finish your Power Yoga program is Savasana, often known as the Corpse pose. Savasana promotes muscular relaxation and protects against injury.

Other Power Yoga poses that are crucial for weight reduction are Uttanpadasana, also known as the posture with raised feet, Veerbhadrasana, the warrior pose, Ardha Chandrasana, also known as the half-moon pose, and Paschimottasana, also known as the stance with bent knees while seated. An effective method for weight reduction and preventing obesity is power yoga.

Conclusion

Yoga, an ancient Indian technique for rejuvenation of the mind and body, offers many advantages for everyone, from those who are overweight and wish to lose weight to those who just want to unwind.

Yoga not only supports weight reduction but also a healthy balance of the body and mind.
Yoga, an age-old healing practice, has outstanding therapeutic potential. Yoga may be very beneficial for your overall health and well-being. While some individuals vouch for the health advantages of yoga, others are a bit dubious about its effectiveness in helping people

lose weight. However, they both agree that yoga, when used in conjunction with diet and nutrition, may help someone lose weight. Keep in mind that your yoga practice is unique to you. It's crucial to maintain proper posture while doing yoga asana, which may be accomplished with effort and repetition.